Ongoing Records Review

A Guide to JCAHO Compliance and Best Practice

Jean S. Clark, RRA

OPUS COMMUNICATIONS
A Division of *hc*Pro

Ongoing Records Review: A Guide to JCAHO Compliance and Best Practice is published by Opus Communications.

ISBN 1-57839-038-9

Opus Communications is the publishing division of HCPro, which provides information resources for the healthcare industry. Opus Communications and HCPro are not affiliated in any way with the Joint Commission on Accreditation of Healthcare Organizations.

Jennifer I. Cofer, Executive Publisher
Rob Stuart, Publisher
Kristen Woods, Executive Editor
Jean Clark, Author
John Devins, Editor
Jean St. Pierre, Art Director
Mike Mirabello, Graphic Artist
Thomas Philbrook, Cover Designer

Advice given is general. Readers should consult professional counsel for specific legal, ethical, or clinical questions.

For more information on this or other Opus Communications publications, contact:

Opus Communications
PO Box 1168
Marblehead, MA 01945
Telephone: 800/650-6787 or 781/639-1872
Fax: 800/639-8511 or 781/639-2982
E-mail: customer_service@opuscomm.com

**Visit Opus Communications and HCPro on the World Wide Web:
www.hcpro.com, www.hcmarketplace.com, www.himinfo.com**

TABLE OF CONTENTS

ABOUT THE AUTHOR

Jean S. Clark, RRA, is currently Director of Health Information Services at CareAlliance Health Services in Charleston, South Carolina. She is past president of the American Health Information Management Association (AHIMA) and the Quality Management Section of AHIMA. She is also currently a director on the executive board of the International Federation of Health Records Organizations (IFHRO), serves as a member of the Joint Commission on Accreditation of Healthcare Organizations' Professional and Technical Advisory Committee for Hospitals. Mrs. Clark is the author of "International Opportunities," from A *Career Guide for Health Information Management Professionals*, published by PRG Publishing, Inc., 1997.

PREFACE

In January 1998, the Joint Commission on Accreditation of Healthcare Organizations (JCAHO) revised its standards regarding medical records review and completion, requiring that these functions be conducted on an ongoing basis. Health information professionals actually provided input into the revision that gives healthcare organizations more flexibility in developing their records review processes. Even though the revised standards seem as straightforward as the old clinical pertinence review requirements, the same questions remain: How do you perform this function in an effective and timely way, and how do you encourage physicians to complete their records?

The new standards provide an opportunity for innovation, as healthcare facilities turn what has often been a cumbersome paper process into a streamlined records review system that is integrated into existing PI programs. We emphasize the importance of involving physicians in the records review process and of fostering a collaborative atmosphere that will improve patient care and increase the overall efficiency of the facility.

Our goal in creating this practical guidebook is to give readers a clear-cut explanation of the revised JCAHO standards and a step-by-step guide to developing an ongoing records review program that best suits the needs of your facility. We break down the main elements of ongoing records review and provide example charts and forms from successful ongoing records review programs. Two in-depth case studies in Chapter Seven present the experiences of different hospitals in implementing ongoing records review programs.

We hope that this book provides readers with a much broader understanding of ongoing records review processes and practices and of the many opportunities for positive organizational change afforded by the revised JCAHO standards.

CHAPTER ONE

Understanding Ongoing Records Review and the JCAHO Requirements

Introduction: Clearing up the confusion

In 1998, the Joint Commission on Accreditation of Healthcare Organizations (JCAHO) revised its standards pertaining to medical records review to focus on a continuous, or ongoing, process; the JCAHO calls this process *ongoing records review*. Before this, records review was mandated quarterly and was known as *clinical pertinence review*. Although the JCAHO has only two standards pertaining to ongoing records review, IM.3.2.1 and IM.3.2.1.1, there is considerable confusion among healthcare facilities as to what these few standards actually require, and how best to demonstrate compliance with the standards.

The confusion stems mainly from not knowing what is meant by the new term "ongoing." Should records be reviewed daily, weekly, monthly, or bimonthly to meet this requirement? The answer could be any of these. The JCAHO standards do not state how or how often reviews should be done. As long as a facility is using a performance improvement approach to ongoing records review—that is, a planned and systematic approach to reviewing records, trending findings to identify opportunities for improvement, taking action as needed, and conducting follow-up—the ongoing requirement will be met.

The main changes

The JCAHO's revised standards have shifted their focus in several main areas:

- Ongoing, rather than quarterly, review of medical records is required. This less-prescriptive approach allows for greater leeway in developing individual records review processes.

- There should now be a continuous performance improvement approach to reviewing the completeness and timeliness of information documented in medical records. As in any performance improvement activity, when problems are identified, staff conducting records review should take action to improve the quality and timeliness of documentation and then follow up on this regularly to assure continued compliance.

- Concurrent, point-of-care reviews are emphasized over retrospective reviews after discharge. Even if a physician dictates a thorough history and physical, if it is done a week or two after discharge, that information is not available when needed for patient care.

- Facilities are no longer required to review at least one record for every physician, but must review a sample of records representing the medical practitioners and the care provided at the facility.

The new standards provide flexibility for the individual facility in developing a systematic and effective approach to identifying opportunities for improvement. Facilities now have a greater choice about how often they conduct medical records review, what criteria they use, and the methodology they employ. The JCAHO believes these changes will make the records review process ultimately more effective. All of this does not mean, however, that the role of the health information manager in the process will diminish. In fact, as the following chapters will show, the revised standards provide an opportunity for the health information manager to serve as a facilitator for the program, rather than the person who must perform the less than gratifying task of reviewing closed records.

How this book will help

Since an understanding of the JCAHO's standards is the foundation of an effective ongoing records review program, this first chapter looks in detail at the JCAHO's standards and their accompanying intent statement and scoring guidelines. But because the JCAHO standards are only a starting point in understanding ongoing records review, the remaining chapters of the book discuss in detail the essential activities of and the decisions involved in setting up an ongoing records review program. They outline the necessary steps for complying with the JCAHO's standards and present many different ongoing records review activities— from selecting review teams, topics, and criteria to presenting evidence of improvement to JCAHO surveyors.

The standards explained

Facilities must review the presence, timeliness, legibility, and authentication of certain data and information, as appropriate to the facility's needs (see Figure 1.1 for the JCAHO standards). At a minimum, the review process must be conducted by the medical staff, nursing personnel, and other relevant clinical professionals as appropriate to the focus of the review.

Figure 1.1

JCAHO Standards for Ongoing Records Review

IM.3.2.1: Medical records are reviewed on an ongoing basis for completeness and timeliness of information, and action is taken to improve the quality and timeliness of documentation that impacts patient care.

IM.3.2.1.1: A representative sample of records is included in the review process.

Source: *1998 Comprehensive Accreditation Manual for Hospitals*, JCAHO, Oakbrook Terrace, IL.

The records review process must be ongoing and cover all clinical areas where care is provided. This should include physicians' offices if they are part of the facility's organization. Findings from ongoing records review must be available for review—at least quarterly—by the group, team, or committee with responsibility for ongoing records review. Who receives this report will depend on your facility's reporting structure; it could go to a medical executive committee (MEC), a performance improvement (PI) committee, or another such group or individual with responsibility for oversight of ongoing records review.

Scoring for IM.3.2.1

To score a 1 on the areas covered by standard IM.3.2.1, a facility must show that it has a process in place to ensure that there is complete and timely documentation, as appropriate to the facility's needs. The 19 items (or those applicable to your facility) listed in the intent statement (see Figure 1.2) should be reviewed some time during the review process. This does not mean that a facility has to review all 19 items

Figure 1.2

The JCAHO expects a review of medical records to address the following, as appropriate to the organization's needs:

- Identification data;
- Medical history, including the chief complaint; details of the present illness; relevant past, social, and family histories (appropriate to the patient's age); and an inventory by body system;
- A summary of the patient's psychosocial needs, as appropriate to the patient's age;
- A report of relevant physical examinations;
- A statement on the conclusions or impressions drawn from the admission history and physical examination;
- A statement on the course of action planned for the patient for this episode of care and of its periodic review, as appropriate;
- Diagnostic and therapeutic orders;
- Evidence of appropriate informed consent;
- Clinical observations, including the results of therapy;
- Progress notes made by the medical staff and other authorized staff;
- Consultation reports;
- Reports of operative and other invasive procedures, tests, and their results;
- Reports of any diagnostic and therapeutic procedures, such as pathology and clinical laboratory examinations and radiology and nuclear medicine examinations or treatments;
- Records of donation and receipt of transplants or implants;
- Final diagnosis(es);
- Conclusions at termination of hospitalization;
- Clinical resumes and discharge summaries;
- Discharge instructions to the patient or family; and
- When performed, results of autopsy.

Source: *1998 Comprehensive Accreditation Manual for Hospitals*, JCAHO, Oakbrook Terrace, IL.

---

continually, but rather that it must use these to identify problem areas in documentation and focus on correcting them (see Chapter Three for more information on selecting ongoing records review criteria).

The JCAHO survey team requests evidence of medical records review for the year prior to a hospital's survey date. If a facility can demonstrate findings from ongoing records review for only three out of the four quarters, it will receive a score of 2. A facility will receive a score of 3 if

- medical records are not consistently reviewed on an ongoing basis;

- the findings are available in only two out of the four quarters prior to the survey;

- performance activities to address findings are not evident; and

- the appropriate individuals are not involved in the review.

If findings are available in only one out of four quarters prior to the survey, the facility will receive a score of 4; and if there is no evidence of an ongoing process, the facility will receive a score of 5. Scores of 3, 4, and 5 can result in Type 1 recommendations.

Scoring for IM.3.2.1.1
By requiring a representative sample of records in the review process, the JCAHO is looking for a sample that truly represents the facility's practitioners (though not every practitioner), the full scope of services the facility provides, and the different clinical areas within the facility.

For example, if a hospital owns physician practices, the records from the practices must at some point be included in the ongoing records review program.

For a facility to score a 1 on standard IM.3.2.1.1, it must use a representative sample in its review process. A facility that includes a representative sample in only three, two, or one of four quarters will not receive a score higher than 2, 3, or 4, respectively. If a representative sample is not used, the facility will receive a score of 5. A facility can, if it chooses, review all of its medical records; however, this is not required in the standards and should be considered only if the sample size is too small or if a review of a sample of records indicates that there is a need to review 100% of the records.

Records completion statistics

In addition to the above requirements, the intent of IM.3.2.1 and IM.3.2.1.1 states that medical records completion statistics must be available for at least quarterly review and must be evident in reports regarding this review function. Many facilities monitor records completion through a process separate from their ongoing records review, but facilities should present the results using the same reports and minutes. (See Chapters Four and Five for more discussion on monitoring records completion.)

Important decisions and activities of ongoing records review

Although the above section summarizes the entire contents of the JCAHO standards, intent statement, and scoring guidelines relevant to ongoing records review, complying with the JCAHO and establishing an effective ongoing records review program takes more than just an understanding of the JCAHO requirements. Successful ongoing records review requires well-planned, well-executed activities.

In planning its ongoing records review program, a facility must make the following decisions, presented in no particular order (in different facilities, there may be different groups or individuals responsible for the following decisions):

- how often ongoing records review is carried out (i.e., weekly, monthly, as issues arise);

- which individuals serve on the group responsible for ongoing records review;

- how performance improvement opportunities are identified;

- how and by whom ongoing records review data is gathered (an individual or group usually gathers and summarizes ongoing records review data for the group responsible for the ongoing medical records review program [see Chapter Two for further discussion of this topic]);

- how representative samples of medical records for reviews are gathered;

- which items, or criteria, are reviewed in each medical record;

- how, how often, and to whom the ongoing records review findings are presented; and

- how the facility documents its ongoing records review activities, actions, and improvements for JCAHO survey purposes.

Facilities must also coordinate the above decisions with the planning and execution of the following activities:

- training individuals to serve on the ongoing records review team;

- gathering representative samples of medical records for reviews;

- analyzing items in medical records against the established records review criteria;

- presenting data to the group responsible for oversight of ongoing records review (medical records committee, PI committee, etc.);

- reporting ongoing records review–related findings to appropriate individuals, committees, departments, and other groups;

- planning and implementing performance improvement activities to improve medical records documentation, based upon ongoing records review findings; and

- documenting actions and improvements related to ongoing records review.

The JCAHO provides minimal guidance on the planning and executing of ongoing records review. One of the reasons the JCAHO revised its standards was to allow facilities flexibility in developing ongoing records review programs that meet their particular organizational needs. For this reason, facilities must make the above decisions and plan the above activities themselves. The aim of this book is to provide a clear understanding of the revised JCAHO standards regarding ongoing records review and to give practical guidance in planning and implementing a JCAHO-compliant ongoing records review program.

CHAPTER TWO

Establishing an Ongoing Records Review Team

Introduction

As discussed in Chapter One, although the JCAHO's standards do outline some specific requirements, the changes made to them have, on the whole, allowed for more flexibility, permitting each facility to develop an ongoing records review process that best suits its needs. Existing activities, such as utilization review and the use of clinical pathways, that identify documentation issues should be incorporated into the process when possible. A recent benchmarking survey (see Figure 2.1) conducted by *Medical Records Briefing* indicates that healthcare facilities are changing the way they conduct ongoing records review. Each facility has broad discretion in deciding the who, how, and when of ongoing records review. This chapter presents some ideas on establishing an ongoing records review team and developing successful review processes.

Figure 2.1

Benchmarking Survey—Ongoing Medical Records Review

Have you changed your record review process to comply with the revisions in IM.3.2.1?	Yes - 65%	No - 31%	Unanswered - 4%
How often do you review medical records for completeness and timeliness of information?	Quarterly - 25%	Weekly - 17%	Monthly - 48%
Has the frequency of reviews changed as a result of the revised standard?	Yes - 58%	No - 61%	Unanswered - 1%
What type of records do you pull for medical records reviews?	Discharged patients - 40%	Hospitalized patients - 4%	Combination - 53%
Do you use the JCAHO grid to comply with IM.3.2.1?	Yes - 76%	No - 24%	Unanswered - 1%
Do you use a formal performance improvement approach to resolve problems uncovered during ongoing medical record review?	Yes - 65%	No - 33%	Unanswered - 2%
If you have been surveyed by the JCAHO in 1998, did you receive a Type 1 recommendation for IM.3.2.1?	Yes - 2%	No - 33%	Unanswered - 65%
Do you still review at least one record for every physician?	Yes - 58%	No - 41%	Unanswered - 0%

Source: *Medical Records Briefing*, Opus Communications, Marblehead, MA.

The ongoing records review process can be broken down into four major components:

- identifying the criteria to be reviewed,

- reviewing the records,

- gathering and organizing the data, and

- analyzing the data and taking action as appropriate.

This review process usually involves three groups of professionals:

- the individuals actually reviewing the records,

- the support staff who organize the data, and

- the oversight team or committee that identifies the criteria, analyzes the data, and takes action.

An ongoing records review oversight team typically includes two or three physicians and at least one nurse and one representative from each of the other clinical disciplines. A team with such broad representation will ensure compliance with the JCAHO requirement that a multidisciplinary group oversee the ongoing records review process.

Using established groups for ongoing records review

Because many healthcare facility activities require multidisciplinary review teams, a facility may find that an existing group, team, or committee is well suited to overseeing ongoing records review. Some facilities continue to use the medical records committee for ongoing records review. This committee is already familiar with medical records and already performs activities similar to ongoing records review, such as analyzing medical records for completeness and time-liness (see Figure 2.2 for a sample medical records committee proto-col). The committee's focus, however, should be one of analyzing findings and recommending actions to resolve problems identified in the review process. The ongoing records review oversight function can also be delegated to physician-led groups such as the medical execu-tive committee or the performance improvement committee.

Actual ongoing records review (checking documentation in the charts against established criteria) can be delegated to committees or groups that monitor quality of care, or to clinical departments.

Combining ongoing records review with other review activities

Facilities often combine ongoing records review with other review activities. These other activities may include quality monitoring, analysis of records completion, coding of records, or utilization review. Because the standards' intent is to focus on information at the point of care, facilities should consider combining ongoing records review with other activities that are already in place and that focus on review of open records. An example of this would be to use case managers or utilization reviewers who are already reviewing medical records to determine if the documentation supports the admission and continued stay of patients.

If a facility has implemented clinical pathways, this is an excellent method for incorporating ongoing records review criteria. The

Figure 2.2

Medical Records Committee Protocol

Purpose
The medical records committee will have oversight for the organization's ongoing medical records review program, the review and approval of form and format for the medical record, and any abbreviations used in the medical record.

Scope
Inpatient and outpatient records that include all services provided.

Responsibilities
- coordination and oversight of the organization's ongoing medical records review program
- establishing the calendar for ongoing reviews
- establishing criteria for ongoing medical records reviews
- reviewing records as needed
- analyzing information from ongoing medical records reviews and taking actions as appropriate
- review and approval of form and format for all medical records
- approving abbreviations for use in the medical record
- review, analysis, and action as needed related to monthly delinquent medical records
- other duties as relate to the documentation, use, and storage of medical records within the system

Membership
At a minimum, the membership will be composed of representatives from the medical staff, nursing, health information management, administration, and other clinical departments.

Meetings
Meetings will be held monthly on the second Tuesday in each month at 7:30 a.m.

Reporting
Reports from the committee will be forwarded to the quality improvement committee and the executive committee each quarter.

Statement of confidentiality
All individuals participating on the medical records committee will honor patients' rights to privacy, will protect medical information, and will report information without referring to specific patient names.

facility can have results from clinical pathways that identify documentation problems reported to the ongoing records review oversight committee. Combining ongoing records review with other established processes, when done well, saves time, money, and resources.

Assembling a team specifically for ongoing records review

While some facilities choose to use established committees or combine the function with other reviews, others choose to create a multidisciplinary team specifically for ongoing records review. Creating an ongoing records review team may help draw attention to the importance of ongoing records review and allow a facility to assemble a group of professionals who are interested in and committed to the ongoing records review process.

To be successful, the multidisciplinary team should have the authority to make improvements; and team members must have a clear understanding of the review process, be motivated, and have an interest in effecting change.

HIM director/assistant director as facilitator for the ongoing records review program

However a facility chooses to structure the actual review process, it is important to have only one coordinator overseeing the ongoing records review program. The health information management (HIM) director or assistant director is a good candidate for this position. He or she is familiar with the content of medical records and knows what sources to utilize for review criteria. More importantly, the HIM director or assistant director is an expert in database management and data display. These are important aspects of the ongoing records review process.

Selecting physicians to be team members

Physicians who are willing and able to champion the cause of good documentation are instrumental in the success of the ongoing records review team. It is important to choose physicians who have the respect of their peers and who are interested in and understand the importance of good records documentation. At a minimum, physicians should approve the review criteria, take part in the analysis of the findings, and recommend actions to resolve problems. Whenever possible, physicians should participate in actual record reviews. It is important that those physicians who participate on a review team receive proper recognition for their work.

Physicians' participation in the process will depend in large measure on how efficiently their records review time can be used. Because they are generally too busy to attend a structured team meeting, for example, it is a good idea to have the records they need to review available. A facility should consider designating a place for the records—such as on the units the physician team members frequent the most or in the HIM department; the records should be in the same place from review to review. The criteria review form should be easily visible on the records, and the physicians should be instructed in how to use the form.

Selecting nurses and other clinical professionals

The selection of nurses and other clinical professionals is equally important as the selection of physician team members. A healthcare facility should select individuals who are interested in the ongoing records review process and who, ideally, have been involved in developing forms for their particular specialties and reviewing records for documentation. Staff who have been part of a clinical pathway team or have been performance improvement coordinators are excellent candidates for an ongoing records review team because they are familiar with reviewing records based upon set criteria.

Other team members

Regardless of how a facility conducts the ongoing review of medical records—whether by using an existing committee, a team created specifically for ongoing records review, or a combination of existing review processes—the physicians, nurses, and other clinical professionals involved in the process can spare only a limited amount of time for review activities.

A facility should consider including nonclinical staff as part of the multidisciplinary ongoing records review team. Although the standards no longer identify administrators as required ongoing records review participants, it could be beneficial to include the administrator responsible for the HIM department as a team member. Strategically, it is important for this individual to understand and support the review process. Representatives from the admitting, utilization review, performance improvement, HIM, and IS departments can be useful members of the team as well.

Support staff such as coders or analysis personnel should perform baseline studies at discharge to determine where documentation problems may exist and in what areas the ongoing records review team might conduct focused reviews. For concurrent reviews, HIM staff can provide review forms, help to identify samples of records, and collate the data once the review is done.

Since the JCAHO continues to include the closed medical record review session as part of the triennial survey, the more individuals a facility gets involved and committed to the ongoing records review process, the better. When it comes time for survey, the facility will have its review team prepared to participate in the closed record review session.

Orientation and training of team members

Equally important as selecting ongoing records review team members is the orientation and training of the team. A facility should require team members to attend orientation and training, but should also make it fun. It might serve food and award a certificate of completion to team members who have demonstrated an understanding of the ongoing records review process. A facility should provide team members with a full description of the review process and outline clearly the expectations for attendance and for meeting the goals of ongoing records review. And it should remember that not all team members will know where to find every indicator in the medical record; as members rotate off the team and indicators for review are selected, a facility should develop a schedule for orientating new members and should design refresher courses for remaining members.

Efficient ongoing records review practices

When planning the ongoing records review process, a facility has to take into consideration the schedules of a large number of people— most of whom have limited time and multiple commitments. Thus, providing records in a location that is easily accessible is important, especially if physicians are conducting the actual records review.

The simplest approach to conducting the ongoing records review is to do it concurrently, using simple checklists (see Figures 3.1, page 24, and 3.2, page 25). Scheduling becomes a moot point because team members can review records in the normal course of their work duties.

By combining the ongoing records review process with other types of reviews, such as quality of care, utilization review, clinical pathway processes, nursing, and other clinical department documentation reviews, monthly reviews become more feasible. However, bimonthly reviews or even quarterly reviews may be sufficient, depending upon a facility and its needs.

Reviewing the findings and taking action

The ongoing records review team responsible for overseeing the process should hold monthly or bimonthly meetings to analyze the data collected, identify problems, and take or recommend actions to resolve the problems identified. The ongoing records review team meeting should be scheduled for a set day and time and should not exceed one hour.

CHAPTER THREE

Selecting Review
Topics and Criteria

Introduction

Once a healthcare facility establishes its ongoing records review team,
the team must begin reviewing medical records for completeness and
timeliness of information. This chapter discusses what facilities need
to consider when gathering sample records and developing appropriate criteria for ongoing records review. Although ongoing records
review teams or committees are ultimately responsible for selecting
sample records and criteria, this chapter suggests how other groups
may be involved in these processes.

Because the types of sample medical records, criteria, and responsibilities of ongoing records review vary widely among facilities—there
are many ways of complying with the JCAHO standards—this chapter
is not able to cover all types of systems. Instead, it discusses the main
issues facilities face when structuring their own programs.

Selecting records to review

Though some extremely low-volume facilities are able to review all of their medical records in the ongoing records review process and thus can avoid having to select appropriate samples, most facilities must use samples of records, since reviewing every medical record is neither feasible nor required by the JCAHO. Some facilities review 5% of their total number of records for each monthly review. Other facilities might review all records on selected days of the week, say, Mondays and Fridays. Again, there is flexibility here for an individual facility to develop an ongoing records review process that is best suited to its needs and its administrative structure.

Whatever methodology they employ, facilities that use samples must ensure that the samples represent the practitioners providing care and the care provided. And remember, healthcare facilities are no longer required to review every physician on the medical staff. A facility could consider selecting a sample of its most common diagnoses and procedures, high-risk procedures, and/or a sample of services provided throughout the organization (for example, emergency, outpatient surgery, and inpatient records that include pediatric, obstetrics, surgery, and medical patients). A facility should also include in ongoing records review documentation from other ancillary services such as physical therapy, respiratory therapy, and cardiac rehabilitation. And a facility should include physician office practices in the reviews if the practices are part of the organization.

What are the criteria?

Regardless of whether all records or a sample of records are reviewed to meet the JCAHO standards, facilities must develop appropriate criteria to assess documentation. Ongoing records review must include, at some point, a review of the 19 items listed in the intent of IM.3.2.1 through IM.3.2.1.1 (see Figure 1.2, page 5). The important thing to note here is the qualification, "as appropriate to the organization's needs." Obviously, if the items do not apply to an organization, they cannot be reviewed.

As either a start-up to a new ongoing records review process or as an annual or semiannual exercise, a facility should determine a documentation baseline by reviewing the 19 items in the intent statement. A more intensified analysis of documentation can be accomplished utilizing *Medical Records Briefing's Documentation Guide Special Report*[1] or JCAHO's closed medical record review indicators. At a minimum, a facility should review all the items listed in the quarterly medical records review summary (see Figure 6.1, page 50). A periodic baseline study conducted by the HIM staff—preferably at the time of discharge—will help to identify the documentation issues that should be earmarked for focused reviews (see Figure 3.1 for a sample ongoing records review calendar resulting from a baseline study done in December of each year). The HIM staff should submit the results of the baseline study to the team responsible for ongoing records review so that the team can decide what issues warrant focused review and determine the review schedule.

For example, a baseline review indicates that history and physical reports are not consistently documented on the medical record before surgery and that the ones already charted do not include the basic information. The ongoing records review team conducts a focused review of records prior to surgery being performed. The nursing staff uses a simple check-off form (see Figure 3.2) to review each surgical

---

[1] *Medical Records Briefing*, Opus Communications, P.O. Box 1168, Marblehead, MA 01945.

Figure 3.1

Sample Ongoing Records Review Calendar

Topic	Jan.	Feb.	Mar.	April	May	June	July	Aug.	Sept.	Oct.	Nov.	Dec.	*
Identification data	X											X	The calendar is an example of a planned approach to ongoing records review. A baseline study is conducted in December of each year to determine where documentation problems exist. Beginning in January of each year, focused reviews are conducted on the problem areas. Additional focus reviews may scheduled as other problems are identified.
H&P	X	X	X	X					X			X	
Orders	X											X	
Informed consent	X	X	X	X					X			X	
Clinical obs. including autopsy results				Aut. R.	X	X			X			X	
PN												X	
Consultations												X	
OP notes		X	X	X								X	
Lab, Rad., etc.									X			X	
Organ donations												X	
Final DX												X	
Conclusions at discharge												X	
Discharge summary								X	X	X	X	X	
Discharge instructions												X	
Ad. Dir.			X	X	X				X	X		X	
ER records				X			X			X		X	
Ob. records				X			X			X		X	
Ped. records				X			X					X	
Other													

Figure 3.2

Are the following critical elements present?

Element	Yes	No	Comments
Is the H&P on the chart prior to surgery? If yes, continue.			
Heart exam			
Lung exam			
Mental status			
Exam of body system/part relative to procedure results			
Surgeon's signature			

record. This form remains on the medical record, and at discharge, the HIM director enters the findings in a database. The data is then reported to the team responsible for medical records review, who will decide what action should be taken. Ideally, a performance improvement team would be assembled to recommend action for correction of the problem. The team should include physicians, nurses, transcription staff, and medical record staff.

Review at the point of care

Whenever possible, ongoing review of records should be performed at the point of care and by the caregivers who document in the records. Simple check-off forms such as the ones illustrated in Figures 3.2 and

3.3 can be used to review records. Nurses traditionally perform chart review regularly at the point of care on the units. Other clinical departments do much the same thing. It is important to develop a mechanism to report these review activities on a quarterly basis. The HIM director or assistant director are ideal individuals to facilitate

Figure 3.3

Record Review Checklist—Do Not Remove from Record

Items	Yes	No	NA
ADVANCE DIRECTIVES • Face sheet marked appropriately "Y," "N," "R," "NB," "Peds," "OB" • AD assessment form complete • AD on record, if "Y"			
HISTORY AND PHYSICAL • Recorded within 24 hours of admission • Recorded before surgery			
CONSENT TO SURGERY • Signed by the patient or legal representative			
OPERATIVE REPORT • Recorded immediately after surgery			
VERBAL ORDERS • MD signed VO for restraints, DND, Class II narcotics within 24 hours			
TRANSFUSION • Reason for transfusion documented on blood bank sticker			

this process. It is important to get credit whenever documentation reviews are being conducted, so that a department can more readily demonstrate how it complies with the standards for ongoing records review.

The HIM staff can collate and present the point-of-care review findings to the team responsible for ongoing records review. Information from check-off forms, such as the two examples stated above, should be part of the ongoing records review quarterly report (see Figure 6.7, page 61, for a suggested form for this purpose).

Clinical pathways as a review tool

As mentioned in Chapter Two, clinical pathways can be used as a review tool for identifying documentation problems or as a method to monitor documentation. Indicators such as those noted in Figure 3.4 can be added to the pathway form and checked off by the nurse as part of the daily pathway review. Since documentation is a key component in determining if a critical pathway is being followed, the pathway is oftentimes a good tool to identify documentation opportunities. Figure 3.4 illustrates a performance improvement opportunity identified through the use of a CABG pathway.

As this chapter illustrates, a variety of sources can generate ongoing record review topic ideas. Selection of topics for review can be based upon findings from generic criteria on a random sample of records, recommendations of other teams, known documentation problems, frequent diagnoses and procedures, or facility statistical reports, to name a few. Most importantly, the facility must identify what is useful to the organization, while continuing to meet the JCAHO standards for ongoing records review.

Figure 3.4

CABG Clinical Pathway

Process to improve	Timing of daily weights and lab specimen collection for post-op CABG patients
Team	CABG clinical path team
Problem statement	Department director had 10 patient complaints last month stating that they could not get any rest while in the hospital and were awakened before daylight to be weighed and have lab work done.
Sources of variations	• Surgeons must make rounds between 6 a.m. and 7 a.m., as surgical cases start at 7 a.m. The lab results need to be on the chart consistently by 7 a.m. • The lab reports that 40% of their workload occurs between 5 a.m. and 8 a.m. Many a.m. labs are ordered as "STAT" on a routine basis, which backlogs orders of truly STAT orders. • Patients say that they cannot get back to sleep after the 5 a.m. wake-up. Literature review suggests that timing of weights and routine labs for CABG patients need to be consistent from one 24-hour period to the next for trending; however, there is no clinical significance regarding what time of the day the measurements should be obtained.
Plan improvement	• Physicians order daily weights and routine lab work for 9 p.m. • Protocol for routine weights and routine lab collection to be changed from 5 a.m. to 9 p.m. • Monitor patient and physician complaints for a 60-day trial period. Monitor incidence of lab results on chart by 6 a.m.
Do	January 1
Check	Analysis on March 15 revealed no patient complaints regarding sleep disturbance for weight and labs. No physician complaints regarding absence of lab work on charts for a.m. rounds. Monitoring revealed that 100% of routine labs ordered were on the charts at 6 a.m.
Act	Continue with 9 p.m. weights and routine lab collection time for CABG patients.

CHAPTER FOUR

Using Ongoing Records Review Data to Improve Medical Records Documentation

Introduction

Regardless of who conducts the actual reviews of medical records in an ongoing records review program, it is the responsibility of the ongoing records review team with oversight responsibility to review the data submitted and either act on its findings or recommend actions. The ongoing records review team must also monitor how review information is reported and acted on throughout the health-care facility, and document the final results of all ongoing records reviews. This chapter examines how ongoing records review information is reported and how the ongoing records review team implements improvements and documents results.

Reporting initial findings and identifying problem records

Those responsible for conducting ongoing records review (actually looking in the charts and checking documentation against established criteria) and gathering data should submit reports to the ongoing records review team that include, at a minimum:

- the types of records reviewed (either a random sample or a topic-specific sample),

- the time period from which the records were gathered,

- the names of those who reviewed the records,

- the total number of records reviewed,

- the number of records found in compliance with the criteria, and

- descriptions of problems uncovered, if applicable.

To make the data more useful, the reviewers who collect the data from ongoing records review and prepare the reports should also consider noting the *percentages* of records reviewed that were found in compliance with criteria. For example, learning that 85% of records were in compliance with a criterion may be more helpful than seeing that 121 of 142 records were in compliance.

The ongoing records review team should receive the reports from the reviews in simple, easy-to-read formats. Reviewers should document their results in checklists similar to those used in the actual records reviews, and attach brief notes describing problem areas (see Figure 4.1 for a sample report). Once the team receives the report, it should review the records in question. This review can be done by the entire team or by a designated member, depending on what the findings are; records with physician-related documentation problems should be

Figure 4.1

Summary Report for Records Review

Categories	Q1 Findings	Q2 Findings	Q3 Findings	Q4 Findings	Improvement Initiatives
Identification data	50/50			50/50	100% compliance in Q1. Next review: Q4
Medical history, including • Chief complaint • Details of present illness • Relevant past, social & family histories • Inventory of body system	30/50	40/50	45/50	48/50	60% compliance in Q1 – Problem related to timely H&Ps; interdisciplinary team established to review root causes; problem identified with Dept. of Medicine; dept. chair presented data to April dept. meeting; findings improved in Q2; review monthly.
Summary of the patient's psychosocial needs as appropriate to the patient's age	48/50	50/50	50/50	50/50	96% compliance – Review again in Q3 100% compliance in Q3
Report of relevant physical examinations	30/50	40/50	45/50	48/50	60% compliance in Q1 (See above)
Statement on the conclusions or impressions drawn from the admission history and physical examination	30/50	40/50	45/50	48/50	60% compliance in Q1 (See above)
Statement on the course of action planned for this episode of care and its periodic review, as appropriate	50/50			50/50	100% compliance in Q1. Next review: Q4
Diagnostic and therapeutic orders	50/50			50/50	100% compliance in Q1. Next review: Q4
Evidence of appropriate informed consent	35/50	46/50	50/50	50/50	70% compliance in Q1 – Documentation of risks, benefits, alternatives not found in 35 charts; Medical Record Committee added these elements to new consent form; compliance improved in Q2
Clinical observations, including the results of therapy	50/50			50/50	100% compliance in Q1. Next review: Q4
Progress notes made by the medical staff and other authorized staff	50/50			50/50	100% compliance in Q1. Next review: Q4 100% compliance in Q1. Next review: Q4
Consultations reports if applicable	50/50			50/50	50% compliance in Q1 – Operative
Reports of operative and other invasive procedures, tests, and their results if appropriate	25/50	40/50	50/50	50/50	reports not charted in a timely manner; team with Med. Recs., transcription, and

Figure 4.1 (cont.)

Summary Report for Records Review (cont.)

Categories	Q1 Findings	Q2 Findings	Q3 Findings	Q4 Findings	Initiatives to improve findings
Reports of any diagnostic and therapeutic procedures, such as pathology and clinical laboratory examinations and radiology and nuclear medicine examinations or treatments	30/50	40/50	50/50	50/50	60% compliance in Q; lab reports not on charts in timely manner; Lab developed team and identified issues; corrective actions taken; improvement seen in Q3.
Records of donation and receipt of transplants and/or implants if applicable	50/50			50/50	100% compliance in Q1. Next review: Q4
Final diagnosis(es)	50/50			50/50	100% compliance in Q1. Next review: Q4
Conclusions at termination of hospitalization	50/50			50/50	100% compliance in Q1. Next review: Q4
Clinical resumes and discharge summaries	50/50			50/50	100% compliance in Q1. Next review: Q4
Discharge instructions to the patient and/or family	50/50			50/50	100% compliance in Q1. Next review: Q4
Results of autopsy, when performed	50/50			50/50	100% compliance in Q1. Next review: Q4
Nursing assessment			50/100	98/100	CABG clinical path established in June; 50% of records reviewed on 2S nursing unit did not have assessment for nutritional needs; team with dietary established; criteria to determine need for assessment revised; new form implemented; improvement seen in Q4.
Legibility	20/30	10/25	10/10	15/15	Coders could not read progress notes in one physician's records; Med. Rec. Com. presented data to chairman of physician's dept. who in turned discussed issue with physician; physician compliance improved with use of her PA.

Table, copyright Joint Commission on Accreditation of Healthcare Organizations, 1997. Reprinted with permission. Data provided by the author.

reviewed by physicians, nursing-related problems by nurses, and so on. This second review is important because on occasion, those conducting the actual records reviews may think something in the record is wrong, when it actually is not.

Whatever the findings, it is up to the ongoing records review team to act on them. The reviewers may be asked to clarify certain information in the report, but they are not responsible for implementing improvements.

Documentation problems related to processes

Documentation problems are usually traceable to flawed processes rather than individual errors or omissions. For example, a concurrent records review may reveal that the outpatient surgery records do not always have the history and physical reports documented prior to surgery. This review may also reveal that the reports do not include an examination of the heart, lungs, mental status, and body system related to the procedure. In this case, the ongoing records review team should refer its findings to the surgery department chair for action.

In another instance, a concurrent records review may reveal that referrals for dietary consults are not being documented in records. The ongoing records review team should, having assessed the problem, refer this to the dietary department director for action. The dietary department director should then take a performance improvement approach to discovering the cause or causes of the problem and to coming up with an appropriate solution.

Findings related to individuals

Although, as mentioned above, most records review problems are traceable to flaws in processes, individual physicians or facility employees may occasionally be the source of problems. For example, a physician might not dictate history and physicals in a timely manner. In this case, the team can contact the person responsible directly or refer the findings to the appropriate department director.

Some documentation problems may require medical executive committee (MEC) or even board action. If timely completion of records has been identified as a major problem area, it may take MEC action to impose a stricter policy for records completion.

It is also the MEC's responsibility to decide if findings from ongoing records review, like the issue of timely completion of records, become part of a physician's credentials file. Because records completion is so important to patient care (and to a successful JCAHO survey!), we recommend that this information become a part of the credentials file and be considered at the time of reappointment. Other departments should consider individual findings at each employee's annual evaluation.

Regardless of who ultimately resolves the problems discovered in the course of ongoing records review, it is important that the resulting corrections are reported back to the ongoing records review team, so that, come time for a JCAHO survey, documentation of all ongoing records review activities are assembled in one notebook for easy access.

CHAPTER FIVE

Monitoring Timeliness of Records Completion

Introduction

Timely documentation is critically important to patient care, both during and after treatment. In addition, the JCAHO surveyors give low scores and Type 1 recommendations to facilities that fail to meet basic records completion requirements related to delinquent records. The JCAHO standards and scoring guidelines refer to medical records documentation in well over 150 places. Surveyors look to medical records documentation in the open records with increasing frequency for evidence that the facility carries out its own policies and procedures in the many clinical and administrative areas, including patient rights, patient education, leadership, and the medical staff. This chapter discusses the JCAHO's emphasis on the completion of records and offers guidance and ideas for meeting this ongoing challenge.

Main standards relating to records completion

The following standards suggest that the JCAHO puts a strong emphasis on the timeliness of records completion:

IM.7.6: Requires medical records data and information to be documented in a timely manner. The intent of this standard is to ensure that medical records are completed within 30 days of discharge. The hospital must measure medical records delinquency at regular intervals—no less than quarterly—and report the data as part of the medical records review function.

IM.7.3.2: States that the operative report must be written or dictated immediately after surgery.

IM.5: Addresses the transmission of data and information in a timely and accurate manner.

PE.1.6.1: Requires that each patient's history and physical examination, nursing assessment, and other screening assessments be completed within 24 hours of admission as an inpatient.

Although this is not a complete list of all the JCAHO standards related to timeliness of medical record entries, it does illustrate how review of timeliness is an important aspect of health information management.

Is timely documentation still a problem?

Medical records completion was a recognized problem well before the JCAHO existed. In 1919, when the American College of Surgeons first set minimum standards for hospitals, it included a mandate for accurate and complete records for all patients and defined "complete" much as the JCAHO does today. By 1929, records completion had become a known problem. The Association of Record Librarians of North America, the precursor to the American Health Information Management Association (AHIMA), devoted part of its first annual meeting to the problem of records completion.

In 1995, more than 20% of surveyed hospitals received a score of 3, 4, or 5 on the requirement that medical records must be completed within 30 days of discharge. In 1997, 5.3% of hospitals received a score of 3, 4 or 5 on the requirement that operative reports must be dictated or written immediately after surgery (IM.7.3.2) and on the requirement that when the operative note is not placed in the medical record immediately after surgery, an operative progress note must be entered (IM.7.3.2.2). For IM.7.6, which states that medical records data must be managed in a timely manner, 15.5% of hospitals received a score of 3, 4, or 5.

Other documentation requirements continue to be problematic for healthcare facilities. For example, the documentation of time-limited orders for restraints is a survey focus for 1998 JCAHO random, unannounced surveys.

What has changed?

In 1998, the method used for calculating delinquent records changed, as did the scoring and reporting requirements. One reason for the change was to be more in concert with the intent of IM.3.2—greater focus on open rather than closed records for review. IM.7.6, is the main standard that addresses records completion.

It places the focus is on the hospital's overall delinquent rate and does not include delinquent records for history and physical and operative reports. Although timely documentation of these reports is important and failure to meet the standards can result in Type 1 recommendations, the focus of the review should be the time during which the patient is being treated, not after discharge. Given the pattern of problem areas revealed by baseline reviews, timely documentation and charting of history and physical and operative reports are good focus areas for ongoing records review.

Another change is that you can now include outpatient records in your delinquent rate; just be sure your denominator and numerator match as you calculate your rate. (Note: In Chapter Six, we discuss reporting delinquent records as part of your ongoing records review.)

Administrative support for records completion

Timely records completion depends in large part on a clear medical staff policy that is enforced fairly and without exception; even the clearest policy set by a well-meaning medical staff will be undermined if no one enforces it or if exceptions are allowed. And an unclear policy allows physicians to interpret it however they please. Administration and medical staff leaders must have the fortitude to defend the records completion policy to medical staff members and to enforce it even when such enforcement may be unpleasant.

HIM department

For records completion activities to be successful, it is imperative that the records processing cycle—the time from patient discharge to records completion—be kept as short as possible. This will ensure that incomplete records are available to physicians for a maximum amount of time. Many facilities know they delay in getting their medical staffs records that have to be completed and, therefore, use date of physician availability as the beginning point of their measurement of how long it takes to complete records. Because regulatory agencies and the JCAHO use date of discharge as a beginning point, however, facilities should do the same and should revise their records analysis processes to support the change.

Often, the delay in getting records of discharged patients to physicians for completion is caused by delayed retrieval of applicable records from nursing units. Facilities have instituted various methods to collect records of discharged patients quickly, including having HIM staff make rounds several times daily to pick up records from the different units. Some HIM departments have added records analysis staff to evening shifts so that records can be available to physicians the day after patients are discharged. Other departments have instituted a concurrent process for analysis, which enables the record to be analyzed by the time the patient is discharged.

It is important that HIM departments have computerized systems that allow staff to enter information on what is missing from each record and to track the number and status of incomplete records. Such systems allow the HIM manager to present regular statistics to the oversight committee in charge of monitoring compliance with records requirements.

Physician motivation and support

Another important component of successful records completion programs is motivating physicians. While it is in physicians' best interest to complete records quickly and completely, records completion remains a paperwork chore that takes busy physicians away from their patients. It is important to make the process as easy as possible for the physicians, which means timely charting of transcribed reports and easy access to medical records.

Some hospitals use disincentives to motivate physicians, such as limiting admissions or surgical privileges of physicians with delinquent records. Others use a more positive approach, offering incentives such as food, assistance, and friendly reminders. Figure 5.1 presents some of the many methods hospitals employ to encourage physicians to complete their records.

Perhaps the strongest support for records completion you can have is a physician champion. This may be the chair or leader of the medical records committee or ongoing records review team. The physician champion should be someone who completes his or her records in a timely fashion and has the respect of the medical staff. A physician champion who sets a good example and is not afraid to take a stand and confront his or her peers when necessary can be instrumental in solving the delinquent records dilemma.

Figure 5.1

Methods for Improving Timeliness of Records Completion

Management support

1. As part of the medical records tracking system, produce regular reports showing the number of days after discharge records are completed.

2. Keep basic records completion data on a database. Present that information to the committee/team in charge of medical records timeliness so it has an ongoing look at completion cycles. Implement a computerized tracking system.

3. Present such information graphically; it's generally more meaningful to the committee.

4. Compare delinquency percentages to patient volume so offenders stand out.

5. Provide an area for physicians to complete records that is pleasant. Clean up! Paint! Try not to have stacks of records lying around!

6. Send records needing to be signed to physicians via courier service, or fax reports. If physicians don't sign the reports in two days, discontinue the service.

7. Use physician extenders to dictate histories and physicals, with the attending physician countersigning them within 24 hours.

8. If physicians don't complete their discharge summaries on time, have a resident complete the documentation and send the physician a bill for the time.

9. Find out what physicians prefer—the specific days and times most convenient to them for records completion. Then tell each physician the department can have the incomplete records ready at his or her preferred time. All physicians are not equal! Determine what works for each one and use it!

10. Ask physicians to call the HIM department a few minutes or hours before they plan to complete records. That way, the staff can have records ready for the physician.

11. Establish a rule that all incomplete records must remain in the department (exception: patient care). If incomplete records are needed for other reasons, such as quality review, staff must come to the department to review them.

Figure 5.1 (cont.)

Methods for Improving Timeliness of Records Completion (cont.)

12. During concurrent review, before flagging a record for a missing report, check the dictation system to find out whether it's been dictated.

13. Assign different colored stickers to each physician. Then, as staff review records for completion, they signal missing items by the color unique to the physician responsible.

14. Use color coding—red is especially noticeable—to indicate documents that need immediate signing, such as operative reports.

15. On admission, put a records completion checklist on the front of the chart and have everyone who puts any documentation in the record indicate when that's accomplished. That eliminates work for the HIM department after the patient is discharged and makes missing elements obvious to the attending physician.

16. Make sure every physician has equal access to records after discharge. The system of putting records in one physician's file until he or she completes them, then moving them to the next physician's file, and the next, simply doesn't work. It's better to file records by terminal digit or in numerical order so all physicians have equal access to them.

17. Go to the nursing unit to retrieve records of discharged patients instead of waiting for them to arrive in the HIM department.

18. Create satellite areas on nursing units where records staff consolidate incomplete records.

19. Rotate staff who do deficiency analysis with those who help the physicians with records completion—it gives both groups a better appreciation of the physicians' problems.

20. Have unit staff assemble the record as much as possible at patient discharge. The HIM staff can simply add transcribed or late documents, thus more quickly getting records to the physician for completion. Better yet, institute a "universal" chart order, and don't reassemble after discharge.

Figure 5.1 (cont.)

Methods for Improving Timeliness of Records Completion (cont.)

21. Have evening clerks on the units or in the HIM department assemble, analyze, and file the day's discharges so the records are ready the next morning for the physicians.

22. Make sure someone who is cross-trained in record completion policies is available to the physicians at all times.

Administrative support

23. Make sure records completion statistics are part of the consideration for recredentialing each physician.

24. Create and enforce a time frame shorter than 30 days for records completion. A requirement of 15 days, for example, gives 15 extra days for the hospital to make sure all items are completed.

25. It's basic, but hospital administration as well as medical staff leaders have to uphold the requirements for medical record completion. And they must apply them to every physician because making exceptions sends the message that the hospital is not serious about records completion.

26. Make sure the president of the medical staff or another person whom physicians respect stresses—at every opportunity—the value of timely records completion, what is required of physicians for records completion, and the process for completion.

27. To reduce the number of unsigned verbal orders, reduce the number of verbal orders taken by restricting them to emergencies only. Define "emergency."

28. Work with other hospitals in the system or in the city to make records completion requirements—including disincentives—consistent across all hospitals. Thus, physicians lose the threat of taking their business elsewhere.

29. Have the HIM department call the physicians with delinquent records.

30. Add a part-time position of physician liaison to the staff and make follow-up on delinquent records his or her responsibility.

Figure 5.1 (cont.)

Methods for Improving Timeliness of Records Completion (cont.)

31. Have the vice president of medical affairs call the department chairs of delinquent surgeons to tell them to cancel their surgeries until records are complete.

32. Don't allow delinquent physicians to preregister patients for admissions or schedule surgeries. Apply the policy to both inpatients and outpatients.

Physician motivation

33. Hold "dine and sign" lunches.

34. Make speaker-phones available to physicians dictating in the HIM department. When using them, physicians have their hands free to shuffle pages in the medical records.

35. Help physicians make the most of their time in the HIM department by separating the records that need signing from the ones that need dictation.

36. Notify the medical executive committee about any physicians that are on the suspension list for three consecutive times. Require the physician to come before the executive committee to explain his or her reasons for delinquent records. Put a copy in the credentials file.

37. Keep several hand-held dictation units available for physicians to borrow for dictation in their cars or when they are away from a phone.

38. Help out surgeons and anesthesiologists by taking all their incomplete records to the physicians' area in the recovery room. Even better, monitor the surgery schedule, and if a physician with incomplete records is scheduled to do surgery, take his or her records to the operating room lounge.

39. Establish a "mini" chart room in the obstetrical lounge so the obstetricians can complete records while waiting for mothers to deliver.

40. Take incomplete records to physicians when they gather for medical staff committee meetings, continuing education meetings, and staff meetings.

Figure 5.1(cont.)

Methods for Improving Timeliness of Records Completion (cont.)

41. Take records to the physicians' lounge or surgery records to the surgery lounge for completion between operations.

42. Use food as an enticement. Managers use all sorts of goodies to encourage physicians to come to the HIM department, from cookies, candy, popcorn, and coffee to continental breakfasts and even weekly lunches.

43. Remember that some physicians are colorblind; if that's the case, use striped tags to ensure they can readily locate their required documentation.

44. Identify medical staff members who miss signing documents and offer to have staff review their records as they are being completed.

45. Hold a contest for residents to see who dictates the most discharge summaries on the day of discharge.

46. Rather than suspending the admitting privileges for one physician, suspend them for the physicians' entire group.

47. If there are several hospitals in a system, suspend the physician at all of the hospitals.

48. Keep up with records delinquencies by clinical department, and increase or decrease the budget yearly based on records performance.

49. Publicize, through bulletin boards or medical staff newsletters, the names of physicians who complete their records on time or the names of the worst offenders.

50. Fine residents who fail to complete records on time. Or withhold their paychecks until they complete records. Tougher still: Make each resident complete all his or her records before allowing him or her to graduate.

51. Use physician pressure on residents. Assign the job of policing medical records completion to the chief of service rather than to residents. Or suspend the admitting physician along with the resident when a record is delinquent. Or

Figure 5.1 (cont.)

Methods for Improving Timeliness of Records Completion (cont.)

institute a policy that if the resident has not signed a record within so many days, the record becomes the responsibility of the attending physician.

52. Suspend other needed services when physicians have delinquent records, such as providing copies of dictated reports that physicians need for billing.

53. Give physicians who have incomplete records personal treatment by calling their offices to alert them and by offering staff help as they complete records.

54. While many disincentives and incentives work, a survey *Medical Records Briefing* conducted several years ago showed that rapport with physicians was second only to suspension of privileges in its effectiveness.

55. Use interdepartmental mail or couriers to hand-deliver notices of incomplete records or delinquent records.

56. Put notices of incomplete records or delinquent records on brightly colored stationery and envelopes so they stand out from the physicians' regular mail.

57. When the physician signs on to any hospital computer, program the screen to flash if any records are incomplete. Or give a list of physicians with delinquent records to the front office of the hospital and ask staff to notify the HIM department when the physicians come in.

58. Use humor. A cartoon or poem sent with the notices of incomplete or delinquent records may get attention when a severe warning does not.

59. After records are incomplete for several days, send a reminder to the physicians every week. And send a weekly list of physicians with delinquent records to their department chairs.

60. Use quality improvement tools to determine why records aren't complete. Don't assume that records are incomplete simply because physicians hate to do them. Instead, look more deeply at the problem to determine whether forms need redesigning, physicians need reeducating, or equipment causes more obstacles than it corrects. Make sure the HIM department's processes are efficient and timely!

Figure 5.1(cont.)

Methods for Improving Timeliness of Records Completion (cont.)

61. Many hospitals find the number of forms has grown out of control. A review of the forms in use will likely find many that are unwieldy, redundant, or confusing. Fewer, better-designed forms may facilitate records completion. Ask for physician input in the process of reviewing, reducing, and redesigning forms.

62. Use electronic signatures software for signing reports.

63. Reduce the number of items you require for record completion, if state and federal laws allow.

64. Give residents a discount on meals when they meet records completion requirements.

65. Post a list of records over three months old that are unbillable due to incompletion.

CHAPTER SIX

Demonstrating Compliance to JCAHO Surveyors

Introduction

While this book has, up to this point, discussed how healthcare facilities should conduct ongoing records review, it is also necessary for facilities to be able to demonstrate good ongoing records review programs to JCAHO surveyors. As part of the documents review and the closed medical record interview, JCAHO surveyors will want to see the documents that reflect ongoing review of records and the outcomes and actions related to these processes. They will also want to see the JCAHO Medical Record Review Summary Sheet (see Figure 6.1) as well as the Medical Record Statistics Form (see Figure 6.2, page 52). This chapter discusses documents that will help facilities organize their ongoing records review programs and monitor performance improvement, while providing the documentation necessary for a successful JCAHO survey.

Figure 6.1

2000 Medical Record Review Summary Sheet

The following items are required (IM.3.2.1–IM.3.2.1.1) to be included as part of the organizations ongoing review of medical records. The review must address the **completeness and timeliness of information** of the items listed. While the review is expected to be ongoing in nature, at least quarterly findings for the review process should be available and activities to address improvement evident. This form, once completed, will be used by the surveyors to orient them to the scope of the medical record review activities of your organization for the twelve months prior to survey. The Completed form should be attached to the medical record review material supplied for the Document Review Session (the document review session is a survey activity designed to prepare and orient the surveyors for subsequent survey activities). Such material should include reports or minutes for the twelve months prior to survey of the group responsible for the review of medical records.

Were the following items included in the review of medical records during the twelve months prior to survey?	Findings (Numerator/Denominator)				Performance improvement initiative to address findings if appropriate
	Q 1	Q 2	Q 3	Q 4	
Identification data					
Medical history, including: • chief complaint • details of present illness • relevant past, social, and family histories • inventory by body system					
Summary of the patient's psychosocial needs as appropriate to the patient's age					
Report of relevant physical examinations					

Were the following items included in the review of medical records during the twelve months prior to survey?	Findings (Numerator/Denominator)				Performance improvement initiative to address findings if appropriate
	Q 1	Q 2	Q 3	Q 4	
Statement on the conclusions or impressions drawn from the admission history and physical examination					
Statement on the course of action planned for this episode of care and its periodic review, as appropriate					
Diagnostic and therapeutic orders					
Evidence of appropriate informed consent					
Clinical observations, including the results of therapy					
Progress notes made by the medical staff and other authorized staff					

Figure 6.1 (cont.)

2000 Medical Record Review Summary Sheet (cont.)

Were the following items included in the review of medical records during the twelve months prior to survey?	Findings (Numerator/Denominator)				Performance improvement initiative to address findings if appropriate
	Q 1	Q 2	Q 3	Q 4	
Consultations reports if applicable					
Reports of operative and other invasive procedures, tests, and their results if appropriate					
Reports of any diagnostic and therapeutic procedures, such as pathology and clinical laboratory examinations and radiology and nuclear medicine examinations or treatments					
Records of donation and receipt of transplants and/or implants if applicable					
Final diagnosis(es)					
Conclusions at termination of hospitalization					

Were the following items included in the review of medical records during the twelve months prior to survey?	Findings (Numerator/Denominator)				Performance improvement initiative to address findings if appropriate
	Q 1	Q 2	Q 3	Q 4	
Clinical resumes and discharge summaries					
Discharge instructions to the patient and/or family					
Results of autopsy, when performed					

©Joint Commission on Accreditation of Healthcare Organizations, 1999. Reprinted with permission.

Figure 6.2

2000 HAS Medical Record Statistics Form

Organization/ID: _____

City/State _____ Full _____ FOC _____ CONF/U _____ SPL _____

Overall Statistics/Organizational Timeframe:

1. Average Monthly Discharge Rate (AMD): _____

Total number of inpatient discharges in the 12 months prior to survey ÷ 12

*Note: This number represents all inpatient discharges (**and can include other records such as** observation beds, ambulatory surgery, endoscopy, cardiac catheterization, or emergency department*).*

*The records included for delinquency counts should be included in both the numerator and denominator of the calculations.

2. Medical Record Delinquency Timeframe: _____

As specified in the medical staff rules and regs. (See footnote 1.)

Quarterly Measure:

3. Total Medical Record Delinquency Rate

Please see note at end of this document that refers to HCFA timeframes.

For each quarter prior to survey, note the **average medical record delinquency rate.** (See footnote 2.) This includes records delinquent *for any reason*.

TOTAL AVERAGE = total of all quarterly averages ÷ 4.

Note: The total average is compared to the AMD listed in 1. above

Quarter 1 Average	Quarter 2 Average	Quarter 3 Average	Quarter 4 Average	TOTAL AVERAGE

Figure 6.2 (cont.)

2000 HAS Medical Record Statistics Form (cont.)

Important Notes

- Type 1 recommendations will be made for medical record delinquency if the total average for total medical record delinquency (documented in 3. above) exceeds 50% of the AMD.

- If the total medical record delinquency rate is equal to or exceeds twice the average monthly discharge rate (AMD), conditional accreditation will be recommended at the time of survey.

- It is important to note that some HCFA timeframe and authentication requirements are more stringent than those of the Joint Commission. If a HCFA validation survey were conducted following a Joint Commission survey and the organization complied only with Joint Commission requirements, a deficiency may be cited by HCFA.

Completed by

_____(Print)_____ Date: _____
Name/Job Title

_____(Print) _____ Date: _____
Name/Job Title

Footnotes:

[1] If the medical staff has not defined a timeframe or if it exceeds 30 days, the value entered here should reflect the number of complete charts (not single components) still open 30 days post-discharge for any reason.

[2] For example: an organization calculates medical record delinquencies on the last day of every month. If the organization's triennial survey starts on December 15, total the raw medical record delinquency counts for November, October, and September and divide by 3. Enter this quarterly average in the box marked "Quarter 1". Then count back three months (August, July, and June), total those raw numbers, divide by 3 and enter this quarterly average in the box marked "Quarter 2". Continue filling in the remaining boxes in like manner to total 4 quarters or 12 months of data. When all 4 boxes are filled, total all quarterly averages, divide by 4, and enter that calculation in the "TOTAL AVERAGE" box.

©Joint Commission on Accreditation of Healthcare Organizations, 1999. Reprinted with Permission.

Documentation demonstrating ongoing records review (including delinquent record statistics) should be gathered from the year prior to a hospital's JCAHO survey and should be kept together in one place. The HIM director or his or her assistant is usually responsible for compiling in a binder, maintaining, and updating the documentation discussed below.

Ongoing records review policies, procedures, and written plans

Every facility should ensure that its policies and procedures cover the functions of its ongoing records review program. The policies should state the responsibilities of medical staff physicians and the authority of the ongoing records review team. The policies and procedures should clearly indicate the time limits for records completion so that physicians are fully aware of how soon they must complete their medical records.

Facilities should draft written plans for their ongoing records review program that contain the following sections:

- **Purpose:** A brief written statement about the hospital's commitment to assessing medical records documentation.

- **Responsibilities:** A section naming the group or groups responsible for ongoing records review and the functions for which the group(s) are responsible. For example, this section should state that the HIM department gathers data on documentation and presents it to the medical records committee, which reviews the data and either acts directly upon its findings or makes recommendations.

- **Scope:** A section listing which items in the medical records the ongoing records review program covers. At a minimum, this section should include the items the JCAHO requires to be reviewed (see the Medical Record Review Summary Form in Figure 6.1). This section should also include the time requirements for completing each section of the medical record, for example:

  - History and physical examinations must be dictated within 24 hours of admission.

  - Operative reports must be dictated immediately after the procedure.

  - Discharge summaries must be dictated within seven days of discharge and cannot exceed 30 days post-discharge.

- **Topics:** A section stating which types of documentation must be reviewed. Because the JCAHO requires that certain items be included as part of the facility's ongoing records review (see Figure 1.2, page 5), this section should list the items from the Medical Record Review Summary Sheet. If specific diagnoses and procedures are reviewed, these should also be included in this section.

- **Criteria and thresholds:** A separate section (which may be attached as separate sheets to the plan) that lists the specific criteria for items routinely reviewed in the medical records. This section should also indicate a threshold, the minimum number or percentage of records that must be found in compliance with each criterion to avoid intense evaluation. Figure 6.3 provides sample criteria and thresholds for assessing the history and physical section of the medical record.

Figure 6.3

Sample Criteria and Thresholds for History and Physical Examinations

Criterion 1: All patients admitted have a history and physical examination dictated within 24 hours of admission.
Threshold: 100%. A 100% threshold was selected based on the medical staff rules and regulations regarding documentation of history and physicals.

Criterion 2: Obstetrical admissions have a legible copy of attending physician's office prenatal record, except when there is no prenatal care.
Threshold: 100%. A 100% threshold was selected based on the medical staff rules and regulations regarding documentation of obstetric cases.

Criterion 3: Documentation of each history and physical examination contains the following:
  • chief complaint,
  • history of present illness,
  • past medical history,
  • relevant social/family history,
  • review of body systems,
  • physical examination,
  • impression, and
  • planned course of action (can be documented in admission progress notes).
Threshold: 95%. A 95% threshold was selected based on past review of the documentation of history and physicals.

Criterion 4: All surgical patients must have a history and physical examination and a preoperative diagnosis prior to surgery. The only exceptions are emergency cases that note the emergency.
Threshold: 100%. A 100% threshold was selected based on the medical staff rules and regulations regarding documentation prior to a procedure.

Criterion 5: Abbreviations approved by the medical staff are used.
Threshold: 95%. A 95% threshold was selected because it is felt that there will be times when an abbreviation is used before it has been approved for use.

- **Process:** A section describing how ongoing records review data is collected and reported.

- **Action and reporting:** A statement of how the ongoing records review team may act upon its findings and to whom it may report.

- **Statement of confidentiality:** A statement that all those participating in ongoing records review will honor patients' rights to privacy, protect medical information, and report information without referring to specific patient names.

(Note: Facilities may modify or add to the above sections in drafting their plans. Different facilities may also refer to the above sections by different names. Figure 6.4 is a sample ongoing records review plan.)

Forms, minutes, and reports

In addition to its policies, procedures, and written plan, a hospital should also assemble documentation that shows that the plan actually works. Facilities should be able to show examples of criteria evaluated and data gathered in monthly or quarterly reviews. Figures 6.5 and 6.6 (see page 60) show examples of delinquent records statistical reporting.

Facilities should also be able to show JCAHO surveyors that data is evaluated, acted upon, and reported to the appropriate committee. For example, hospitals should assemble the minutes of all ongoing records review team meetings, which reflect ongoing review activities and actions taken to resolve problems. Figure 6.7 (see page 61) is an example of a form that can be used to report quarterly review activities.

Figure 6.4

Ongoing Records Review Plan

Purpose
The organization is committed to assessing, and correcting as needed, the documentation and timely completion of its medical records.

Responsibilities
1. The medical record committee is responsible for establishing review criteria, establishing the annual review calendar, analyzing review findings, taking actions as appropriate, and reporting quarterly to the quality improvement committee and the medical executive committee.

2. Departments, review teams, and HIM department staff are responsible for reviewing medical records against established criteria and reporting findings.

3. The HIM director or his/her designee is responsible for coordinating the overall ongoing records review program. This includes orientation and training and preparing reports for the medical record committee.

Scope
The scope of the ongoing records review program includes both inpatient and outpatient records and all clinical services within the organization.

Topics
Topics include, but are not limited to, the items required by the JCAHO. High-volume, high-risk, and problem-prone areas as well as selected diagnoses and procedures may also be selected.

A baseline of the JCAHO items will be conducted in December of each year to determine the focused reviews for the coming year. However, problem areas may be selected at any time for focused reviews.

Criteria
Appropriate criteria may be selected according to topic by the medical record committee or by the team or department conducting the reviews. The JCAHO accreditation manual is a good source of criteria. At least 5% of records for any topic must be reviewed, or 100%, depending on the sample size.

Figure 6.4 (cont.)

Ongoing Records Review Plan (cont.)

Process
Data collection should be at a the point of care whenever possible. Review of closed records is discouraged. Findings from reviews should be forwarded to the HIM director.

When other documentation review activities such as case management, performance improvement, or clinical pathways identify documentation issues, these should be reported to the HIM director.

Action and reporting
The HIM director will forward findings from all review activities to the medical record committee for action.

Statement of confidentiality
All individuals participating in the ongoing records review program will honor patients' rights to privacy, protect medical information, and report information without referring to specific patient names.

Source: Roper CareAlliance Health Services, Charleston, SC.

Figure 6.5

1998 HAS Medical Record Statistics Form

Overall Statistics/Organizational Timeframe:

1. Average Monthly Discharge Rate (AMD): 2396
2. Medical Record Delinquency Timeframe: 30 days

Quarterly Measure:

3. Total Medical Record Delinquency Rate:

Quarter 1 Average	Quarter 2 Average	Quarter 3 Average	Quarter 4 Average	Total Average
433	566	510	472	495

Figure 6.6

Monthly Delinquent Medical Record Statistics

	JAN	FEB	MAR	APR	MAY	JUN	JUL	AUG	SEP	OCT	NOV	DEC
Monthly discharges	2200	2254	2250	2300	2450	2260	2400	2508	2545	2500	2546	2537
Ambulatory surgery												
DELINQUENT RECORDS	450	375	475	543	468	468	550	525	456	475	485	455
DELINQUENCY <50%	20.45%	16.64%	21.11%	23.61%	28.08%	20.71%	22.92%	20.93%	17.92%	19.00%	19.05%	17.93%

Average number of delinquent inpatient records is <50% of the average monthly discharges (AMD). Average monthly discharges include inpatients, ambulatory surgery patients, and observation patients.

Quarterly statistics												
Total discharges	6704			7010			7453			7583		28753
Total delinquent records	1300			1699			1531			1415		5945
Delinquency rate	19.39%			23.30%			20.54%			18.66%		20.68%

Source: Roper CareAlliance Health Services, Charleston, SC.

Figure 6.7

Quarterly Report—Ongoing Records Review Activities

TOPIC	FINDINGS	ACTION TAKEN
Baseline Study(ies)		
Focus Review(s)		
Concurrent Review(s)		
PI Team(s)		
Delinquent Record Statistics		

Source: Roper CareAlliance Health Services, Charleston, SC.

CHAPTER SEVEN

Case Studies

The following section provides a detailed look at two ongoing records review programs:

- *Crozer-Chester Medical Center, Upland, Pennsylvania*

- *University of California, Irvine Medical Center, Orange, California*

CROZER-CHESTER MEDICAL CENTER
UPLAND, PENNSYLVANIA

For Crozer-Chester Medical Center, what began two years ago as
an initiative to improve reviews of the medical record finished with
the implementation of an ongoing, integrated, multidisciplinary
records review process that drew the praise of JCAHO surveyors.
Raymond Pinder, MS, RRA, director of medical records, along with
Walter L. Bisbee Jr., RRA, assistant director of medical records, and
Debra Harris Lillback, RN, MSN, hospital services quality assessment
(QA) support specialist, were instrumental in developing and implementing the system-wide, standardized medical records review
process at Crozer-Chester.

The new system has proven more effective, efficient, and coordinated
than the previous method of conducting medical record reviews, and
Pinder and his colleagues hope to use it as a model to be put in place
at other facilities in Crozer-Chester's parent organization, the Crozer
Keystone Health System.

Identifying the problem

In anticipation of an upcoming JCAHO survey, the hospital services
QA committee put together an improvement team, led by Bisbee
and Lillback, to coordinate the medical records review process in various departments throughout the hospital. This was a break from the
past, when departments conducted their individual records reviews
without regard to the reviews being done in the other departments.
When Lillback moved from her position as nursing quality assessment

coordinator to the quality monitoring and improvement (QM&I) department, she and Bisbee began to compare the data from the highly individualized departmental clinical pertinence reviews (CPRs) with the more comprehensive data generated by the medical records department's CPRs.

They saw immediately that the data from the two sets of reviews did not match; there were discrepancies in critical areas. The medical records department's CPRs showed omissions in areas that the department's reviews did not identify. Departmental reviews would credit preliminary result reports as being present in charts, whereas the medical records department would identify this as an omission in the closed records review if the final report was not present.

A comparison of the individual departments' data with the data from the medical records department also revealed significant duplication of documentation. Many departments were creating specific forms to facilitate their own documentation processes, which resulted in the same information sometimes being found in numerous chart locations. As a result, medical records staff were spending an inordinate amount of time searching for the information needed to complete their reviews; they were also spending time doing large pulls of records for departments to use in their individual records reviews. In addition, the different forms being created by the different departments led, in some cases, to omissions of documentation.

A decision to make changes

Following the improvement team's assessment of the records review process, Crozer decided to adopt a system of integrated medical records review. The hospital vice president assigned the improvement team the task of coming up with (in six weeks) a complete project plan for the integration of the hospital's departmental documentation reviews with the clinical pertinence reviews done by the medical records department. The team's goal was to eliminate the individual departments' records reviews and replace them with a single multidisciplinary review that would streamline, standardize, and coordinate the entire process.

Developing and implementing a new records review system

The initial step in the project was to train and educate all staff who would be taking part in the new records review process. Every department with responsibility for documentation in the medical records, as well as many ancillary departments, such as pharmacy, occupational therapy, and physical therapy, were asked to send two or three staff members to two two-hour training sessions. These departmental representatives formed the multidisciplinary team responsible for records review. To conduct the training sessions, the team assembled all pertinent medical records documentation forms into a kind of training manual that would be used to illustrate where each criterion is usually documented. By going through each criterion and by addressing all of the departmental representatives' questions concerning the forms, criteria definitions, time frames, and any other pertinent review issues, the improvement team laid the groundwork for a more standardized method of documentation.

The improvement team had to consider the broadest range of standards possible when developing criteria for the integrated medical records review process, so that the final criteria adopted for records review were an assimilation of the individual departments' review processes, the closed record review criteria of the JCAHO, the American Osteopathic Association (AOA) standards, the Commission on Accreditation of Rehabilitation Facilities (CARF) standards, and any relevant Pennsylvania state regulations regarding documentation.

The team likens the new general documentation review forms (see Figures 7.1–7.3, pages 71-73, for sample review forms) to taking an SAT test, where reviewers blacken the circle corresponding to the correct answer—yes, no, or N/A—for a particular criterion. Given this format, a common understanding of definitions is critical. "Yes" and "No" must mean the same thing to everyone for each criterion under review.

How the integrated records review works

Records reviews are done monthly by the multidisciplinary review team. The medical records department also rotates a staff member onto the team—usually a coder or abstractor. The multidisciplinary approach has worked well when reviewing criteria that may have been problematic in the past. With the new records review system, there will always be a representative of the department under question present to answer any questions or concerns regarding documentation methods, criteria, terminology, and so on.

Under the integrated records review system, the team reviews a 5% random sample based on the monthly discharge volume, attempting to review a consistent combination of both inpatient and outpatient records, though this may vary depending on the department. The team lays out a calendar for the year—approved by the medical records committee—such that every major department in the hospital will eventually come under review.

Fine-tuning the review process

Though last year Bisbee and the multidisciplinary review team undertook a comprehensive, full-chart review of every department in the hospital (using the newly created, standardized form with over 100 criteria), the data this generated was deemed more than necessary by JCAHO surveyors, who suggested focused reviews using fewer criteria. As a result, the comprehensive review was segmented into several topic-focused reviews in which about 30 criteria were examined. This has proven much more manageable, says Bisbee.

Last quarter, the team focused its review on the timeliness of documentation:

- Was there a progress note dated, timed, and signed daily?

- Are stat orders—such as for x-rays, medications, or tests—done within the appropriate time frame?

- Is the face sheet completed and dated within 30 days post-discharge by the attending physician?

- Is the nursing admission database completed within the appropriate time frame (eight hours or less)?

Through the use of scanner technology, the data from these focused reviews can be tabulated much faster than before, and the full results can be quickly sent to the medical records committee for assessment. According to Bisbee, scanner technology, combined with more focused and standardized criteria, have given the medical records department the ability to capture this kind of essential data more quickly and effectively. This rapid turnover of data allows the medical records department to spot trends faster and take necessary action, whether preventive or corrective.

For the individual departments, the new system of standardized forms has great appeal. Though created out of an assimilation of criteria from the many departments, the review forms can still produce numbers that reflect what is actually happening in the individual departments.

Follow-up and action when corrections are needed

One of the weaknesses of the previous, nonintegrated medical records review system at Crozer was that it lacked a formalized system for holding individuals and departments accountable for deficiencies in the medical records. Under the new system, the review team reports its findings monthly to both the medical records committee and the hospital services QA committee. If a department falls below the 90th percentile in any criteria, it receives a letter from medical records identifying documentation deficiencies. During quarterly quality monitoring and improvement reports, Lillback checks to see what was done to correct the previously noted documentation deficiencies and follows up as needed. Bisbee regularly attends physician business meetings to report any deficiencies directly to the physicians.

JCAHO survey under the new system

Crozer-Chester was surveyed last January. Pinder reports that JCAHO surveyors were impressed with the hospital's ability to develop and implement an integrated review system in only six weeks and praised the current process. Following the survey, the JCAHO's main suggestion was that more concurrent chart reviews be done so that improvements can be made while a patient is receiving care. Open records review is on Crozer's schedule for next year.

Figure 7.1

General Documentation Review

Discharge Date _____ Medical Record Number _____

Attending Physician Number _____

Scale Definition: 1 = yes 2 = no 3 = N/A	1	2	3
1. Final diagnosis present on face sheet	○	○	○
2. Secondary diagnosis noted on face sheet (Somatic Dysfunction for Osteopathic drs.)	○	○	○
3. Procedures noted on face sheet	○	○	○
4. Advanced directive status noted	○	○	○
5. Copy of advanced directive document present	○	○	○
6. Organ donation status noted	○	○	○
7. Admission consent signed by patient/guardian	○	○	○
8. Overall penmanship of the record is legible	○	○	○
9. Progress note entries signed with credentials	○	○	○
10. Progress note includes OMT (for osteopathic physicians)	○	○	○
11. Progress note entries made by students are countersigned	○	○	○
12. Treatment orders signed with credentials	○	○	○
13. Treatment orders include OMT by osteopathic physicians	○	○	○
14. Treatment orders made by students are countersigned	○	○	○
15. Verbal orders are signed by the physician	○	○	○
16. Entry errors are identified/noted as "error"	○	○	○
17. Errors crossed out by single line	○	○	○
18. Errors are initialed or signed	○	○	○
19. Consult ordering/requesting physician signature on consult sheet	○	○	○
20. Responding or consultant physician signature noted on consult sheet	○	○	○
21. Where home care/equipment services arranged prior to discharge (case mgt. notes time and vendor), there is evidence that freedom of choice was given to patient	○	○	○

Source: Crozer-Chester Medical Center, Upland, PA.

Figure 7.2

Emergency Review

For each item, please select one response by darkening the appropriate circle.

Scale Definition: 1 = yes 2 = no 3 = N/A	1	2	3
1. Evidence of consent for treatment? (Consent Form)	○	○	○
2. Emergency care provided to the patient prior to arrival is documented? (ED Flow Sheet)	○	○	○
3. Upon arrival, triage assessment and prioritization documented? (ED Flow Sheet)	○	○	○
4. Known adverse and allergic drug reactions documented? (ED Flow Sheet)	○	○	○
5. Medications used by the patient noted? (ED Flow Sheet)	○	○	○
6. History of disease and physical findings documented? (ED Record)	○	○	○
7. Age-appropriate assessment documented? (ED Record/ED Flow Sheet)	○	○	○
8. Treatment plan/diagnostic testing ordered and results documented? (ED Record/ED Flow Sheet)	○	○	○
9. If indicated, assessment for abuse/neglect documented? (ED Record/ED Flow Sheet)	○	○	○
10. Diagnosis documented? (ED Record)	○	○	○
11. Physician signature? (ED Record)	○	○	○
12. Final disposition noted? (ED Record/ED Flow Sheet)	○	○	○
13. Condition on discharge documented? (ED Record/ED Flow Sheet)	○	○	○
14. Discharge instructions for follow-up/care? (Discharge Instr. Form)	○	○	○
15. Nursing assessment and reassessment/treatment response? (ED Flow Sheet)	○	○	○
16. Evidence of discussion of treatment plan with patient/family? (ED Record/ED Flow Sheet)	○	○	○
17. Level of care form completed for admitted patients? (Level of Care Form)	○	○	○
18. Documentation of the admitting physician's name/service? (ED Record)	○	○	○
19. All entries, orders, and treatments dated, timed, and signed (with identification)?	○	○	○
20. If emergency report is dictated by physician, is dictation attached?	○	○	○
Documentation of patient transfers (Transfer Form) to other organizations includes:			
21. Reason for transfer?	○	○	○
22. Stability of the patient?	○	○	○
23. Acceptance by the receiving organization (name of physician)?	○	○	○
24. Responsibility during transfer?	○	○	○
25. Copies of relevant patient information/test results sent with the patient?	○	○	○

Source: Crozer-Chester Medical Center, Upland, PA.

Figure 7.3

Obstetrical Review

Please select one response for each item. Additional questions/comments may be noted in comment box.

Scale Definition: 1 = yes 2 = no 3 = N/A	1	2	3
1. Face sheet and stat sheet document infant and maternal ID?	○	○	○
2. Labor and delivery record signed by attending?	○	○	○
3. Delivery note is dated?	○	○	○
4. Delivery note is timed?	○	○	○
5. Delivery note documents the type of delivery (vaginal or C-section)?	○	○	○
6. Delivery note documents the fetal presentation?	○	○	○
7. Delivery note documents if delivery is assisted with forceps and/or vacuum?	○	○	○
8. Delivery note documents the number of pulls (for assisted delivery)?	○	○	○
9. Delivery note documents description of delivery maneuvers used?	○	○	○
10. Delivery note documents type of anesthesia?	○	○	○
11. Delivery note documents condition of the infant?	○	○	○
12. Delivery note documents Apgar scores at 1 and 5 minutes?	○	○	○
13. Delivery note documents infant weight/height?	○	○	○
14. Delivery note documents any complications and/or injuries present at delivery?	○	○	○
15. Delivery note documents description of placenta sample?	○	○	○

Item_____

Item_____

Source: Crozer-Chester Medical Center, Upland, PA.

UNIVERSITY OF CALIFORNIA, IRVINE MEDICAL CENTER ORANGE, CALIFORNIA

UCI Medical Center's transition to ongoing records review began just over two years ago, when the center's financial administrator asked the health information management (HIM) department to build Medicare compliance into its records review process and, if possible, make the reviews concurrent. With this in mind, HIM director Jennifer Hughes and her staff began to assess UCI Medical Center's records review system to see how and where they might revise the system to achieve these goals. The resulting records review system in place at UCI Medical Center not only assures concurrent review, but has the distinction of having anticipated the JCAHO requirement for ongoing records review (standard IM.3.2.1) by nearly two years. The new system has also resulted in a far greater number of staff being involved in and knowledgeable about documentation practices.

Assessing the current system
Soon after finance requested that HIM build Medicare compliance into its records review process, Hughes assessed the whole records review system and decided what changes would be necessary to bring about ongoing, concurrent records review. Concurrence, more than Medicare compliance per se, became the main impetus behind the pending changes.

Up until this point, only a small number of staff were actually involved in the records review process at UCI Medical Center. This group concentrated primarily on physician documentation review, but nursing documentation also needed to be included in the process. If the goal of a concurrent records review system was to be achieved, more staff would have to be involved in the actual reviewing of medical records.

Educating and training reviewers

For there to be coordination and consistency in the records review criteria, terminology, and definitions, Hughes knew that she would have to educate and train the reviewers. Hughes' objective in educating and training a significantly larger core group of records reviewers was to ensure a consistent application of criteria, concurrent review, and a broader staff knowledge of documentation practices and policies. The more staff throughout the hospital who were educated about the importance of good, timely, and accurate documentation, the more concurrent records review would become the norm.

In all, 30 staff members representing all the clinical areas in the hospital participated in the initial training session. Hughes stresses the importance of this full representation as a means of ensuring a system-wide adherence to the established records review criteria. It was essential to establish for the whole group exactly what they would be looking for in their concurrent reviews and where they would find that information in the charts.

With a focus on concurrent reviews, the training fostered a "fix it now" mentality among the core review group. With time, this mentality has spread beyond the core group of 30 records reviewers to any staff throughout the hospital with responsibility for documentation in the medical records. When staff identify a chart element that is missing, inaccurate, or out of place, they act immediately to correct it.

After conducting complete (nonfocused) reviews for approximately twelve months, Hughes came up with a pared-down list of criteria that focused on the high-risk, problem-prone areas of documentation. The group of 30 reviewer-trainees then went over the revised criteria individually to clarify any ambiguous terms and resolve any issues that might lead to varying interpretations of criteria.

The records review group now meets quarterly to discuss the latest review findings, assess how the records review process is working, address any questions that may have come up in the interim, and decide on any actions that must be taken. The group has had several refresher courses since the initial education and training session. Through a kind of trickle-down theory of education and awareness, a far greater number of staff throughout the hospital are in fact more knowledgeable about what is good concurrent medical records documentation. This, says Hughes, is a far cry from the previous system in which a small group of HIM staff did records reviews and reported the findings to a physician committee, at which point the process ended.

The methods of concurrent records review

Records review at UCI Medical Center is done monthly. The majority of the reviewers are nursing staff, but there are also representatives from pharmacy, nutrition services, occupational therapy, performance improvement, and HIM. Each member of the core review group is responsible for reviewing two records per month from his or her area. This is done by taking an arbitrary selection of records, using as a target a 5% sample. Though in a JCAHO survey this past February the process was approved as meeting the "ongoing" requirement, Hughes points out that they are still reviewing only 60 records a month.

Because the core review group is made up of staff from all the clinical areas, the process assures sample records from each area. This alone would ensure that the reviews—in accordance with the JCAHO requirement—included the hospital's full scope of practice. But Hughes has developed a second means of assuring that this requirement is met. For every case she enters in her database, Hughes includes the principal diagnosis, the procedure, the attending physician, and the hospital service. In this way, she can, if necessary, go back retrospectively (Hughes notes that HIM still does some retrospective reviews) to be sure that HIM has reviewed for all UCI Medical Center services and for all physicians.

Focused reviews

Known collectively as Medical Records Documentation Review Criteria (see Figures 7.4, page 81, and 7.5, page 85, for a sample documentation review form and a documentation checklist), the comprehensive criteria form for records review at UCI Medical Center—developed by Hughes using the JCAHO requirements, state requirements, and internal hospital policies as a guide—has 350 different criteria, far too many to obtain focused data on a particular clinical area.

By conducting focused records reviews on individual clinical areas using 25–30 criteria, Hughes is able to obtain more specific data about those clinical areas. If the data reveals deficiencies in the medical record, she can make recommendations for corrective actions.

Hughes and her colleagues decided that, henceforth, focused reviews would be the norm, but that, during one quarter of every year, they would conduct a review using the full 350-criteria checklist. This provides them with an annual comprehensive look at the state of medical records.

How is review data reported?

Every month, each member of the review group forwards his or her data to Hughes, who enters it into a database. In keeping with hospital bylaws, the HIM department reports its findings quarterly to the joint quality and resource management committees (JQRM), the medical staff committee that oversees records review throughout the hospital. HIM also sends a report to the medical staff quality and resource management meetings, so that surgery, medicine, psychiatry, and other departments have an opportunity to review any data relevant to their particular disciplines. These various groups that receive reports from Hughes in turn provide feedback to the records review group. When the process has worked its way full-circle back to the records review group, group members may then, if necessary, make recommendations for changes that the JQRM must approve. Hughes has prepared a document for this purpose known as conclusions, recommendations, actions, evaluations—otherwise known as CRAE. The CRAE document serves as a more formalized means to summarize the main points of the reports and to lay out a plan of action.

The major changes

According to Hughes, one of the more significant changes brought about by the transition to ongoing, concurrent records review is the greatly expanded roles and responsibilities of the records review group. Under the present system, records reviewers are often the primary agents of change and improvement. They are often the first to identify problems in documentation and to initiate discussions about what can be done to correct them. Their job now encompasses far more than what the title "reviewer" might suggest. As the group with the greatest familiarity with the medical records, it is now being asked to come up with solutions to problems.

HIM has implemented concurrent reviews in several places that didn't previously do them. One of those, the post-anesthesia care unit (PACU), now conducts concurrent reviews to ensure that all discharges from that unit are signed off on by a licensed independent practitioner. Reviewers are now checking for this signature *before* patients are discharged.

Physician involvement in the review process

At present, no physicians participate in the actual ongoing records review process at UCI Medical Center; however, because the JCAHO wants them to be part of the process, and because HIM would also like to include them in as many review-related activities and meetings as possible, physicians are brought into the process when specific problems are identified. The physicians chosen to sit in on the last JCAHO survey and participate as part of the special survey review team were those who had demonstrated an active interest in improving medical records documentation.

UCI Medical Center has an incentive reward program that extends to all its employees. Earlier this year, administration decided that if the hospital passed the JCAHO survey with commendation, it would double everybody's incentive reward. This, says Hughes, brought a noticeable improvement in physician commitment to documentation. And, UCI Medical Center's records review process passed its JCAHO survey.

Figure 7.4

UCI Medical Center—Medical Records Documentation Review Criteria

Pt Name: _____

PF#: _____ Attending MD/Svc: _____

Admit Date: _____ Unit: _____

Dsch Date: _____ Diagnosis/Proc: _____

Reviewer: _____ Date of Review: _____

Emergency Care Provided by UCI:		Y	N	N/A	Comments
1. Time and means of arrival documented	Emergency room record				
2. Conclusions at termination of treatment include final disposition	Emergency room record; if patient left AMA, that must be specified				
3. Condition at discharge documented	Emergency room record				
4. Instructions for follow-up care documented	Emergency room record				
5. Faculty signature present on emergency department medical record	Emergency room record				
6. Order sheet completed	Emergency room record-order sheet				
7. Attending note present	Emergency room record				
8. Resident signature included	Emergency room record				
9. Medications/IV fluids administered have an order	Emergency room record				
10. Vital signs documented including B/P (B/P if age>3 years only)	Emergency room record				
11. Weight documented (only applicable on patients <=15 years of age)	Emergency room record				
12. Diagnosis appropriately written	Emergency room record				

Figure 7.4 (cont.)

UCI Medical Center—Medical Records Documentation Review Criteria (cont.)

Emergency Care Provided by UCI:		Y	N	N/A	Comments
13. Reason for transfer documented, when applicable	Patient Transfer form				
14. If transferred, stability of patient documented	Patient Transfer form				
15. If transferred, acceptance by receiving organization	Patient Transfer form				
16. If transferred, responsibility during transfer noted	Patient Transfer form				
17. If transferred, relevant info. went with patient	Patient Transfer form				
History and Physical:					
1. On record w/in 24 hrs. (or if done w/in 7 days before admission, an interval note is also present)	Date on hand-written H&P; date of dictation/filing on typed H&P				
2. Chief complaint	History and Physical				
3. Details of present illness	History and Physical				
4. Family history	History and Physical				
5. Psychosocial history	History and Physical				
6. Review of systems	History and Physical				
7. Physical exam includes breast, rectum, pelvic	History and Physical				
8. Impression/diagnosis	History and Physical				
9. Treatment plan	History and Physical				
10. Mental status eval & DSM IV for Axis 1–5 (Psychiatry)	History and Physical				
Assessment:					
1. Physical status assessed	Nursing Admission Assessment or on the body systems section of the flowsheets				
2. Psychological status assessed	History and Physical or Nursing Admission Assessment or Clinical Social Work assessment (either on PR or CSW)				

Figure 7.4 (cont.)

UCI Medical Center—Medical Records Documentation Review Criteria (cont.)

Assessment:		Y	N	N/A	Comments
3. Social status assessed	Nursing Admission Assessment or Clinical Social Work assessment (either on PR or CSW) or physician history and physical				
4. Nursing assessment completed in accordance with policy	Date/time on Nursing Admission Assessment compared to patient arrival time on flowsheet				
5. Nutrition screen completed	Nursing Admission Assessment— Nutrition/Metabolic section				
6. Nutritional status assessed, when warranted, in compliance with Nutrition Screening/Assessment Criteria	Contact your dietitian for collaborative review; progress notes (blue notes)— refer to Nutrition Screening/ Assessment Criteria for timeliness guidelines				
7. Functional status assessed	Nursing Admission Assessment—Activity/ Exercise section				
8. Functional assessment performed for each rehab referral	Psychiatrist form				
9. Need for discharge planning assessed	Nursing Admission Assessment— Discharge Planning section				
Progress Notes Present and Include:					
1. Clinical observation and results of therapy	Progress notes (blue notes)				

Figure 7.4 (cont.)

UCI Medical Center—Medical Records Documentation Review Criteria (cont.)

Progress Notes Present and Include:		Y	N	N/A	Comments
2. Significant lab, x-ray, other diagnostic tests and/or therapeutic procedures	Progress notes (blue notes)				
3. The effectiveness of medications for the patient is continually monitored	PR (Patient Record), flowsheets, vital signs sheets				
4. Physician communication with healthcare providers	Progress notes (blue notes), Consultation report				
5. Periodic review of treatment plan	Progress notes (blue notes)				
6. Patient's progress is periodically evaluated against goals and the plan of care	PR (Patient Record), Progress notes (blue notes)				
7. Attending note present per bylaws	An entry in the blue notes—*EACH DAY*				

Source: UCI Medical Center, Orange, CA.

Figure 7.5

Medical Records Documentation Checklist

Reviewer's Name: _____

Date : _____

	YES	NO
H&P/Assessment/Reassessment	❏	❏
H&P is dated within 7 days of admission; interval note required if >24 hours old	❏	❏
H&P on chart within 24 hours of admission or prior to surgery (if sooner)	❏	❏
H&P is signed by the attending physician	❏	❏
Nursing admission assessment is COMPLETED within 24 hours of admission	❏	❏
Admission form into PR TDS within 24 hours	❏	❏
Assessment includes:		
Nutrition screen (PR TDS)	❏	❏
Functional screen (PR TDS)	❏	❏
Barriers to education	❏	❏
Religious values (PR TDS or Form)	❏	❏
Cultural values (PR TDS or Form)	❏	❏
If patient has advance directive, either a copy is in the record or patient's wishes are documented in the record (PR TDS and Open Plan)	❏	❏
Response to and effectiveness of medication is documented for all PRN meds (for pain management: assessment documented within 24 hrs; response documented within one hour)	❏	❏

Orders

	YES	NO
All verbal orders are signed within 48 hours except for orders for restraint/seclusion, which must be signed within 24 hours (ORD TDS printout)	❏	❏

Figure 7.5 (cont.)

Medical Records Documentation Checklist (cont.)

	YES	NO
All orders for restraint/seclusion note reason for restraint, and are time-limited to 24 hours (no PRN orders are acceptable [ORD TDS/Order Form])	❏	❏
All orders are timed (Physician Order Sheet)	❏	❏

Operative Cases

	YES	NO
Brief op note in progress notes is written immediately following surgery (consent/blue notes)	❏	❏
Pre-op checklist indicates pre-op teaching is completed	❏	❏
Typed operative report is signed by attending surgeon (within 72 hours following surgery)	❏	❏
PACU discharge is written by attending anesthesiologist	❏	❏

Interdisciplinary Plan

	YES	NO
Interdisciplinary plan of care is appropriate to patient's current condition	❏	❏
Interdisciplinary teaching plan is present, current/documented on (TDS or Form)	❏	❏
Barriers to education are assessed with each teaching interaction (Teaching Plan/blue notes)	❏	❏
M.D. notes reflect education of the patient/family (blue notes)	❏	❏

DNR Charts

	YES	NO
There is a note that indicates there was a discussion with the patient's family regarding DNR status and the wishes of the patient/family are respected (PR TDS & Open Plan)	❏	❏

Charts of Patients in Final Stage of Life
There is evidence in the chart of the following:

	YES	NO
Comfort (symptomatic) management	❏	❏

Figure 7.5 (cont.)

Medical Records Documentation Checklist (cont.)

	YES	NO
Pain management	❏	❏
Psychosocial support	❏	❏
Spiritual needs	❏	❏
Emotional needs	❏	❏
Involvement of patient	❏	❏
Involvement of family, as appropriate	❏	❏

General

	YES	NO
There is a daily progress note by the attending physician	❏	❏
All entries are dated, timed, and authenticated with title of entrant (blue notes/R1, R2, R3, A)	❏	❏
Informed consents are legible, completely filled in, and signed	❏	❏
Attending physician's signature is found on all informed consents	❏	❏
Medical students' blue notes are co-signed	❏	❏
Advance directive status has been determined and upgraded within 48 hours if it is a 4 (PR)	❏	❏
Blood transfusion physician has discussed with the patient/family the outcomes and alternatives regarding such treatment (consent/blue notes)	❏	❏

Source: UCI Medical Center, Orange, CA.

CONTINUING EDUCATION QUIZ

Complete the quiz by clearly writing the letter corresponding to the correct choice for each question on the answer sheet found on the last page. If you expect more than one person to take the quiz, photocopy the answer sheet and use the copy to record your responses. The answers to each question can be found in the chapters of *Ongoing Records Review: A Guide to JCAHO Compliance and Best Practice*. You may refer to the chapters as you take the quiz.

Send only the answer sheet(s) back to us with a $30 payment for each person who completes the quiz. (All quizzes must be prepaid. Checks should be made payable to *Opus Communications*). To qualify for the three hours of CE credit, you must get 75% of the answers correct—that's 23 out of 30 questions.

We'll send you a certificate of completion that you may use for display and for documentation of your CE hours for the American Health Information Management Association (AHIMA).

This program has been granted approval by the American Health Information Management Association (AHIMA) for three continuing education hours. It satisfies the requirements of the Clinical Data Management (CDM) core educational content area. Granting prior approval in no way constitutes endorsement by AHIMA of the program content or the program sponsor.

Chapter 1

1. The JCAHO requires that healthcare facilities review medical
    records on an ongoing basis.
    a. true
    b. false

2. To score a 1 on the JCAHO standards relating to ongoing records
    review, a facility must review a representative sample of records
    a. in three of four quarters.
    b. in two of four quarters.
    c. in one of four quarters.
    d. in four of four quarters.

3. A facility must review at least one medical record from each
    medical staff physician per month.
    a. true
    b. false

4. Which professionals should compose the group responsible for
    ongoing records review?
    a. physicians
    b. nurses
    c. other clinical professionals
    d. all of the above

5. All 19 items listed in the intent statement of IM.3.2.1 through
    IM.3.2.1.1 must be reviewed for the presence, timeliness,
    legibility, and authentication of the data.
    a. true
    b. false

Chapter 2

6. The team responsible for ongoing records review is charged with
    a. reviewing the medical records against established criteria.
    b. developing clinical pathways based on the findings of records review.
    c. comparing the appropriateness of treatments and procedures against established clinical guidelines.
    d. analyzing findings from the medical records reviews and implementing actions, recommendations, and improvements.

7. Which of the following groups may perform ongoing records review?
    a. the medical records committee
    b. the performance improvement committee
    c. a multidisciplinary team
    d. all of the above

8. Which of the following is important when selecting the physician members of the ongoing records review team?
    a. physicians who never miss a meeting
    b. physicians who are interested in and understand the importance of good records documentation
    c. physicians who are frequently on the suspension list
    d. physicians who get along well with their peers

9. Support staff may be selected from the following:
    a. utilization reviewers
    b. health information professionals
    c. performance improvement staff
    d   all of the above

10. Ongoing records review must be conducted separately from other types of reviews.
    a. true
    b. false

Chapter 3

11. Random samples of records may be used for all of a healthcare facility's medical records reviews.
    a. true
    b. false

12. Random samples of records should include
    a. the most frequent diagnoses and procedures.
    b. high-risk procedures.
    c. all services provided.
    d. all of the above

13. A good way to identify focus reviews is to conduct a baseline study using the 19 items, as appropriate, in the intent statement of IM.3.2.1 through IM.3.2.1.1.
    a. true
    b. false

14. The JCAHO standards encourage medical records review after discharge.
    a. true
    b. false

15. The following groups are good sources for ongoing records review topics.
    a. safety committee, performance improvement committee, governing board
    b. pathway teams, performance improvement teams, medical record committee
    c. both a and b

Chapter 4

16. The initial report submitted by those responsible for reviewing records and gathering data should **not** include
    a. the types of records reviewed.
    b. the time period from which the records were gathered.
    c. the number of records found in compliance with the criteria.
    d. the patients' names in the records reviewed.

17. A second review of medical records by the ongoing records review oversight team may be necessary.
    a. true
    b. false

18. Generally, documentation problems in ongoing records review are traceable to the review processes being used.
    a. true
    b. false

19. Results of ongoing records review must be reported at least
    a. bimonthly.
    b. quarterly.
    c. monthly.
    d. annually.

20. Problems related to the medical staff should be reported to the
    a. board.
    b. performance improvement committee.
    c. medical executive committee.
    d. none of the above

Chapter 5

21. The JCAHO is not concerned with timely completion of medical records.
    a. true
    b. false

22. The JCAHO requires facilities to track the timely completion of records for
    a. overall delinquent records, delinquent records due to history and physical reports, and delinquent records due to operative reports.
    b. overall delinquent records.
    c. delinquent records due to history and physical reports and operative reports.
    d. unsigned reports.

23. The JCAHO does not allow outpatients to be included in the delinquency rate.
    a. true
    b. false

24. Facilities should use _____ as the beginning point of their measurement of how long it takes to complete medical records.
    a. date of discharge
    b. date of records availability
    c. date of completion of the discharge summary
    d. none of the above

25. All disincentives or punishments are ineffective in motivating physicians to complete medical records.
    a. true
    b. false

Chapter 6

26. Ongoing medical records review documentation helps facilities
    a. keep better records.
    b. demonstrate compliance with JCAHO standards.
    c. track review of invasive and other procedures.
    d. none of the above

27. Documentation demonstrating ongoing records review and delinquent records statistics should be made available to the JCAHO surveyors.
    a. true
    b. false

28. Written ongoing records review plans do not typically contain which of the following?
    a. responsibilities of groups and individuals
    b. the scope stating which items in the medical records the ongoing records review program covers
    c. a list of the physicians and departments with known documentation problems
    d. the criteria and thresholds

29. A facility should be able to demonstrate that its ongoing medical records review program identifies and resolves problems.
    a. true
    b. false

30. Usually, the HIM director or assistant director is responsible for maintaining and compiling the documentation demonstrating a facility's ongoing records review program.
    a. true
    b. false

ANSWER SHEET

We suggest that you photocopy this page and use the copy for your responses. Please write the letter corresponding to the correct answer next to the question numbers below.

Chapter 1	Chapter 2	Chapter 3	Chapter 4	Chapter 5	Chapter 6
1. _____	6. _____	11. _____	16. _____	21. _____	26. _____
2. _____	7. _____	12. _____	17. _____	22. _____	27. _____
3. _____	8. _____	13. _____	18. _____	23. _____	28. _____
4. _____	9. _____	14. _____	19. _____	24. _____	29. _____
5. _____	10. _____	15. _____	20. _____	25. _____	30. _____

Check one:
❏ ART ❏ RRA ❏ Other (please specify) _____

Name _____
Telephone _____
Address _____
City _____ State _____ Zip _____
AHIMA (AMRA) ID # _____

Please enclose a $30 check payable to Opus Communications for each individual answer sheet submitted. Mail to:

Opus Communications
P.O. Box 1168
Marblehead, MA 01945